2013 Medicare Advantage?

D. I. Stevenson

Copyright © 2012 D. I. Stevenson

All rights reserved.

Cover Image: Amanda Mills 2011

ISBN-13: **978-1480205321**
ISBN-10: 148020532X

DEDICATION

Dedicated to my grandparents Pete & Donna, without them and their generation, there would be no Medicare.

CONTENTS

	Acknowledgments	i
1	Important Facts & Information	3
2	Election Periods	6
3	5 Stars	8
4	Health Coverage	9
5	Prescription Coverage	12
6	Resources	14
7	Checklist of Questions	15

ACKNOWLEDGMENTS

This book is designed to be easy to navigate, answer basic questions you may have as well as provide a checklist of questions to ask when dealing with any sales agent.

This book will be especially advantageous to children of those individuals just becoming eligible for Medicare for the first time. I recommend getting the answers to those questions in this checklist for multiple plans, then decide which is right for you or someone close to you.

In the spirit of disclosure I have 3 years experience working inside of a Medicare Advantage organization. I have seen the ins and outs of what should have happened prior to a member choosing are particular Medicare Advantage plans. Each plan is different and will fit a variety of needs, so prioritize, filter, and select a plan.

1 IMPORTANT FACTS & INFORMATION

For the sake of this book we will assume that you or a loved one already meets the criteria to qualify for Medicare. Traditional Medicare is split into three basic parts, Part A, Part B, and Part D. The ID card for Traditional Medicare is commonly referred to as your "Red, White, & Blue" card. If you do not carry a Medicare Advantage Plan, or do not have other private primary insurance, this is your health insurance card.

Part A: typically covers Hospital Care, Nursing Facilities, Hospice, and Home Healthcare Services.

Part B: typically covers the rest of your medical needs such as durable medical equipment, outpatient services for mental healthcare, some outpatient prescription drugs, and preventative services typically carried out by a standard specialist (think dermatologist) or your primary care physician (PCP for short).

Part D: you are required to carry a form of prescription drug coverage, this is done through private companies, some Medicare Advantage Plans combine parts A, B, & D to keep things simple for consumers, but not all plans do.

Part C: combines your Medicare Part A & B into a single option, more commonly known as Medicare Advantage. As previously stated some Medicare Advantage plans will also include Part D, some do not. If the plan you choose does not, you are required to select one separately for your prescription coverage.

Medicare Advantage Plan Types:

Health Maintenance Organization (HMO): this plan type accounts for the majority of the Medicare Advantage Plans on the market today, and has a very similar set up to general private insurance plans. There are co-pays, deductibles, coinsurance, and most importantly a Provider Network. In some cases out of network doctors are covered at 0% which can become a disaster if this were to go unchecked. You are also required to have a Primary Care Physician (PCP) on your account at all times, you are typically able to change it freely. However, make sure in advance your primary doctor accepts your new insurance.

Regional Preferred Provider Organization (PPO): this plan type opens the provider network to entire states or regions, with the idea that it opens up rural areas to more access to Medicare Advantage plans. This plan type functions much in the same way as an HMO but is limited in scope geographically. You do not typically need to maintain a PCP on file, but may pay more money to see non-preferred doctors.

Other key Terms & Definitions:

Primary Care Physician (PCP): your primary family doctor, used as a gatekeeper for referrals, health maintenance visits, prescriptions, authorizations, and care.

Referral: a prescription from your doctor to see a specialist or for durable medical equipment (think cane or wheelchair). Some plans require these, some do not so be careful.

Authorization: an authorization is typically reserved for more expensive services, and are above and beyond a referral. They typically require your health care provider to submit records that support their requesting the specific test or equipment.

Formulary: the list of drugs that your prescription drug plan will cover, not all plans are the same, so checking to make sure your favorite medications are covered is key. There are specific medications that are Medicare Part D Excluded medications, that is the federal government does not allow Part D plans to provide these specific types of medication. (One example from 2012 was Xanax which is part of the benzodiazepine therapeutic class).

Co-pay: a flat fee paid for products or services, an example would be a $20 fee every time you would visit your PCP.

Co-insurance: this is the Traditional Medicare form of payment, what it means is that you as a consumer would pay 20% of the doctor's fee or equipment price based on the Medicare negotiated rate. A simple example would be as follows: You go to see a neurologist for a screening, that neurologist charges Medicare $400 for that visit. Medicare has a negotiated rate of $200, so they send the doctor a payment of $160 (80%), and that doctor would in turn bill you for the remaining $40 (20%). The biggest downside is no cost assurance as medical billing can become full of add on charges that could run that $40 bill into the hundreds.

Deductable: the amount of out of pocket expenses you must incur prior to your coverage "kicking in" and paying their share.

Premium: the monthly fee you pay for your services, some Medicare Advantage plans take only the premium Traditional Medicare removes from your social security check, while others charge a premium amount above that.

Provider: another name for doctor or vendor providing services or materials.

Coverage Gap: or more commonly known as the "Donut Hole" is a limit imposed by your Part D plan, that kicks in after you and your plan combined have spent $2,930 on prescriptions for the year. Your out of pocket expenses increase dramatically until you have spent a total $4,700 out of pocket for the year, before coming back down to a reasonable level.

Even more detail can be found at http://www.medicare.gov

2 ENROLLMENT PERIODS

There are a host of enrollment periods that apply to Medicare recipients, and it can get confusing to know which applies to Medicare Advantage. I will do my best to help you stay informed.

If you do not currently have any Medicare Coverage and will coming due for Medicare Eligibility you will qualify for what is known as the Initial Enrollment Period, allowing you to select and enroll into a plan up 3 months prior to the month you become eligible, during that month, and up to three months after. But waiting until the last minute could result in a delay.

The Open Enrollment period is for individuals currently enrolled in a Medicare Plan of any type that may be looking for a change. The dates vary slightly from year to year but typically run between October 15th and December 7th with changes taking effect the first of the following year. This is open season, and anyone eligible for Medicare will be bombarded with advertisements, mailers, commercials, and letters. We will soon be helping you cut through that fat and get to the meat of Medicare Advantage.

If you found yourself with buyer's remorse following the Open Enrollment period there are some ways out, some specific to only certain situations while others are there for everyone to enjoy. My goal is to give the masses as much info as they can use and in as few pages as possible, so we will keep the special cases to a minimum.

General Enrollment Period can be taken advantage of between Jan 1-Feb 28, allowing those individuals who signed up for a Medicare Advantage plan the opportunity to switch back to Traditional Medicare only, taking effect the first of the following month after they decided to leave their Medicare Advantage plan. Everyone can take advantage of this one.

Special Election Periods apply to specific situations and allow individuals to switch between Traditional Medicare, Medicare Advantage Plans, and back again. Some cases that allow for this include moving to a different coverage area, changes that cause you to lose your other coverage, changes in your plan, and a host of other special cases. If you think your case qualifies contact 1-800-Medicare to confirm.

My personal favorite, and the topic of its own chapter is the 5 Star enrollment period. Simply put, the best of the best Medicare Advantage plans are labeled as 5 Star Plans. You can choose to switch from you current plan into a 5 Star Plan at any time between December 8-November 30th. Plans range between 1-5 stars and can be used to gauge a plans overall levels of effectiveness.

3 5-STAR PLANS

We briefly discussed 5 Star Plans in the Enrollment Periods. In this chapter we will discuss how the Star Rating is determined and how it pertains to you.

The Five-Star Quality Rating System is operated through the Center for Medicare and Medicaid Services. The idea behind it is to help quickly educate consumers on what it is that they were buying into. It even requires plans to clearly label themselves in terms of their star rating. The five domains measured are as follows:

a) Screenings and preventive tests: the plans ability to get their members to receive routine screenings and exams as a means to keep high cost procedures at bay.

b) Managing chronic conditions: how the plans help members get through tough conditions such as cancer.

c) The total number of member complaints that come through the plan and the total level of members that leave the plan. This centers around the plan being able to come through when it says it is going to.

d) Overall plan responsiveness or their ability to get their members care within a timely period.

e) Customer Service, ultimately tied to a variety of variables, but gives an accurate description of the type of service you would expect from your health organization.

Here is some insider knowledge that they will not tell you when attempting to sell you a 5 star plan. Medicare, being the giant organization that it is, does not assign star ratings based on same year data and feedback. In fact the star ratings you will see for 2013 are a result of data, feedback, and audits from 2010. Essentially just because a plan is labeled as 5 star, does not mean they are currently operating at a 5 star level, just that they did. Asking the right questions is key to getting each plan to stand alone on its own merits currently, not just its Star Rating.

4 HEALTH COVERAGE

Medicare requires that each Medicare Advantage plan to cover at the bare minimum what Traditional Medicare provides in terms of products and services. There is no limit to the additional products and services that a Medicare Advantage plan can provide. This is how they attempt to differentiate themselves from plan to plan.

Here is a short list of items and services that Traditional Medicare does not cover but you may find on various Medicare Advantage plans.

- Dental care of any type, including dentures which many seniors find themselves in need of before it's all said and done.
- Glasses and contacts
- Chiropractic (routine)
- Routine transportation
- Over the counter items such as adult diapers
- Gym memberships

The cost per service listed above vary depending on the organization, but each item should be prioritized, depending on your budget you may be forced to choose between one or another. I highly recommend starting with an open mind and narrowing your choices from there.

Some of the tricks you will see within these organizations stem from co-pays, coinsurance, service limits, and authorization requirements. For example, on a skilled nursing facility stay in 2013 Medicare would charge $0 for days 1-20, then $144.50 per day for days 21-100. An advantage plan may charge $500 per day for days 1-10, then $0 a day after that. What they neglect to say is that typically an individual will get downgraded from a skilled nursing facility to either home health care or a lower level of care within a very short period of time, so the insurance company essentially make sure they are getting all of their co-pays without "dragging it out" to 100 days.

Some additional items to look out for with ancillary benefits such as vision and dental. For vision, does it cover glasses? How often? Does it cover no line bifocals, transitional lenses, eye exam, diabetic eye exam, cataract surgery, more glasses after surgery, how much do they charge per visit? For dental, is there a separate deductable, what is the coverage limit per year? Does it cover full dentures or just partial dentures? Hearing aids, does it allow for both ears in one year, or simply one ear, what is the co-pay, and how often can I get another hearing aid? Is there a limit on routine transportation? Is there a co-pay, is the limit one way trips or round trips?

As you can see just from these few short pages that there is a lot to look at prior to moving from Medicare to a Medicare Advantage plan. And do not forget the number one most common "issue" that plagues a Medicare Advantage Member - their network. Always make sure the provider you want to use, regardless of the service, accepts the Medicare Advantage plan that you choose.

An example scenario that is more common than you would think, you contact a specialist provider (think dermatologist) and ask if they take "Insurance X". The receptionist says, well of course we take "Insurance X". You have your visit and 6 weeks later your receive a large bill for the provider not being in network. You call the office and they apologize. They did not realize it was the Medicare Advantage form of "Insurance X". Always be specific with the type of plan you have when talking with providers and save yourself some hassles.

If you are someone that is in need of special recurring treatment of any health condition, you want to make sure it is not something that needs to be authorized in advance of the plan covering it. It is a play on words, but an item can be "covered" by the plan, but may require "Authorization" prior to the plan agreeing to pay for it. This could result in a delay of service or unwanted bills.

This brings us to our next topic, non covered benefits.

Medicare requires that each Medicare Advantage plan at least review requests from you or your provider for services that are not covered by the plan. The Medicare term for this is called an Organization Determination, and is typically applied for by your provider. These requests have to be investigated and decided on by health professionals. They are open for appeal if denied. It is better stated in the following example.

Suppose you, as a member, would like lipo-suction surgery, and it is not a covered benefit. However, both you and your provider feel it would be life changing. You can contact your health plan and put in a formal request for it to be covered. If they deny it, you can appeal that decision. If they deny the appeal, you can actually appeal to an independent review board, which can overrule the health plan. In other words, the sky is the limit for requests, and these organizations are required by law to hear you and your doctor out.

And your ultimate weapon against any case that you feel was mishandled is called a grievance. A grievance can take on many forms. The ones that effect a health plan the most, and they spend the most money trying to prevent, is the CTM Complaint. CTM stands for Complaint Tracking Module and logs the number of complaints a health plan receives through either 1-800-Medicare or congressional offices. These are directly tied to the 5-star ratings discussed earlier so you are not powerless in scenarios that do not end up going your way.

*One additional warning, there are specific services called preventative services. They include things such as mammograms and colonoscopies. You will often see them listed as "Free". Make sure you clarify whether or not they stay free if and when something shows up in these exams. Let me offer an example, if a colonoscopy turns up a polyp, it may change from a routine (free) screening to a diagnostic procedure in terms of billing. This could mean thousands of dollars, so look for plain clear type that these are free regardless of the test out come.

5. PRESCRIPTION COVERAGE

Medicare requires that every member carry some sort of "credible coverage" for prescription drugs. This can be through an employer or outside organization, however be careful as there are penalties for each month that you do not carry "credible coverage" while you have Medicare. It is in an attempt to spread the cost of prescriptions around versus just joining and cancelling plans as you need prescriptions. The late enrollment penalty is a complicated topic and is best researched outside of this book. Simply ensure you have an active prescription drug plan from the time you join Medicare. And if you are unsure whether or not your plan qualifies, contact Medicare directly at 1-800-Medicare or 1-800-633-4227.

Let's assume that you will be choosing your Part-D prescription drug plan at the same time you are joining a Medicare Advantage plan. As stated previously in the book, there are options to select an Advantage Plan that already comes equipped with a drug plan or shop for one separately. I highly recommend the former as it is easier to keep track of contacts, plan specific processes, and customer service activities. However each choice should be made on individual wants and needs, so let's discuss what to look out for.

Part D excluded medications, do not confuse these with non formulary medications which a health plan chooses not to cover. These are medications that Medicare states cannot be covered. There are numerous examples and vary year to year. Some of the most common that cause members a lot of grief are anxiety medications (2012), erectile dysfunction medication, and for those that are disabled and still young enough for child bearing, birth control. These should not vary by plan, so go in assuming these will not be available.

The formulary is what will set each plan apart from the other And it should be stated that these formularies must include all drugs that will treat the conditions that Medicare requires be treated. This does not however have to be the same brands as offered by Traditional Medicare. For example Atorvastatin is a generic name for Lipitor, which a plan may cover. Another plan will also cover Atorvastatin but may do so in the form Crestor. Be sure you are clear if you require brand specific medication.

Each plan is different but they typically separate their drugs into tiered categories. The higher the tier, the higher the co-pay. It is wise, whenever the co-pay is equal to or greater than the retail pharmacy price, to make sure you pay cash and do not charge to your insurance. This will help delay your entry into the "coverage gap".

Similar to medical coverage you want to make sure that your local pharmacy participates with your new insurance plan. The transfer can cause unnecessary delays in you getting your covered medications on time. There are two other items to look into besides if the medication is covered. Similar to medical services, does it require special authorization? This has to be offered by each plan, and is typically applied for by your prescribing provider. If denied, there is a similar appeal process mandated to be available to you. The other fine print item to check is if there is a quantity limit per month, common amongst pain relievers, and is best discussed up front to prevent any delay in prescriptions when changing plans. Many plans offer a one month transitional refill to provide a window of opportunity to settle any authorization requests (Coverage Determinations). What they will leave out however, is that one month supply will typically be at the cost of their highest tier for non specialty medications. So be weary that if all of your medications require authorizations, month number 1 may be quite pricey.

We will cover resources available to you in our next chapter followed by the step by step questions to help narrow down the plan right for you.

6 RESOURCES AVAILABLE

Each plan will have their current year summary of benefits available to you online and during an in-person sales visit, so I will not link to those here. What I will point you to are some great online resources for general and specific plan information.

Help With Medicare Costs:

http://www.medicare.gov helps point you to a variety of sources, such as state Medicaid Programs, Savings Programs, PACE, and Supplemental Social Security Income. 1-800-Medicare can also point you in the right direction.

Prescription Drug Help:

You may qualify for a Low Income Subsidy (LIS) for prescription drugs which would limit you to a fixed co-pay, or small coinsurance, and the best part is anyone who qualifies for LIS will never end up in the "donut-hole". http://www.ssa.gov or 1-800-772-1213 to apply.

General Medicare Information:

1-800-Medicare: you can find out who in your area offers a Medicare Advantage Plan, what their ratings are, and what your current levels of coverage are.

http://www.medicare.gov : contains a treasure trove of knowledge about everything you ever wanted to know about Traditional Medicare. It also contains some important forms that would need to be filled out if you plan on someone helping you keep up on your medical affairs.

http://www.cms.gov : The Centers for Medicare and Medicaid Services is the overseeing body of Medicare Advantage, a great resource if you have not had your fill after reading Medicare.gov.

The Henry J. Kaiser Family Foundation: http://www.kff.org spends a lot of time and money providing one of the best sites on the internet for Medicare information.

7 MEDICARE ADVANTAGE CHECKLIST

If you are still with me, and I hope that you are, it is in this recap that I hope to save you from some potentially damaging errors when choosing the right Medicare Advantage Plan for you.

1) Write out a list of your doctors, hospitals, facilities, and pharmacies that you visit on a regular basis. Which of these doctors would take the new version of your insurance (remember to reiterate to office staff that this is the Medicare Advantage version)? Are there any doctors on this list you could potentially live without if you had to select a different specialist?

2) Write out a list of the current prescriptions you are taking and what you currently pay out of pocket for those medications. Are you taking the brand name or the generic? Does your doctor feel like an alternative to your specific brand of prescription would be of no consequence (this could mean a lot of savings)? Is there a quantity limit on the specific medications that you are on?

3) What are the co-pays or co-insurance associated with your most commonly used items and services? Focus on these first. Is there a limit to the number of items/visits/uses of each service you listed? Do any of them require a prior authorization before you could continue these services?

4) What does this plan have in place for emergency services? Long term services? Inpatient care and skilled nursing facilities? Remember that some co-pays are front loaded heavily to capture as much guaranteed cash as possible.

5) Are preventative services actually free? Remember the colonoscopy example from above?

6) Double check whether or not you qualify for any of the additional financial help that is listed above. It never hurts to check and the pay offs can be huge.

7) Outline a list of benefits or services that you would love to see on a plan, as this should help narrow the field considerable. I highly recommend

placing an emphasis on medical and dental services over vision care as vision care can typically be had for relatively small costs in comparison to dental and medical services.

8) What is the price? Focus on premium (monthly fee), and deductable (out of pocket expenses before your insurance kicks in).

9) Use this opportunity to remove some of your plan options based on the criteria above. Assuming you have a couple left that meet or exceed your needs as a consumer, let their service set the them apart.

10) Daily customer service check, gather up a few standard benefit questions you have had come up during your research, call the individual health plans and ask the questions. This should give you a feel for this plan and how it will respond if you truly needed assistance. For a true indicator of customer service, call mid-day on a Tuesday or Wednesday. Friday afternoon will have the lowest hold time, but you really want to know how these plans operate at their busiest time.

11) Look for any special nurse lines, case management, or incentives. Some plans go to the extreme to get you into your preventative services. It is not uncommon to find gift cards, transportation, or free over the counter items as incentive.

Remember these key items when selecting a plan:

1) Whether it is covered or not Medicare requires health plans to allow you to request just about any item or prescription you choose, and if the plan denies this request they have to allow you to appeal.

2) Do not be afraid to switch plans if yours ends up not working as well as it should. Within your first month you should know if you made the right choice.

3) If you are not sure if a product or service is covered, always contact the plan directly. They have the most knowledge about your own specific item or service as it pertains to their benefits.

4) No matter what a salesperson tells you, a Medicare Advantage Plan is a REPLACEMENT to Medicare, not a SUPPLEMENT, meaning the Advantage plan will become your insurance, and your Medicare card would not be used unless you went back to Traditional Medicare. There are plenty of supplemental plans that work with Traditional Medicare, they are a breed

all of their own and are best described by someone other than myself. Good luck on your quest to finding the Medicare Advantage Plan that is right for you or your loved one.

It is always smart to consult a professional when dealing with things as complicated as insurance, but I personally believe in being as well informed prior to entering those types of transactions. Thank you for taking the time to read this short book and I hope it has helped.

The opinions in this book were that of my own and do not reflect those of any commercial entity. The websites listed in the resources section are 100% owned and copyrighted by their prospective parties and were in no way affiliated with this book. Insert chapter seven text here.

ABOUT THE AUTHOR

As written earlier in this book I am an employee within a Medicare Advantage organization, one of the largest in the country. I published this book under a pseudonym to ensure I keep my job. I have a background in business and finance and enjoyed writing this book. I care deeply for the individuals in this country that require Medicare in any form and only hope to provide some guidance within the foggy atmosphere of insurance.

This is my first book and is of course self published. With any luck there will be a second!

www.ingramcontent.com/pod-product-compliance
Lightning Source LLC
Chambersburg PA
CBHW061523180526
45171CB00001B/306